The

Mindful

Eater

A Step-by-step Guide by

Dr Lebo

Published by

Afroshapers

The Mindful Eater

Copyright © 2023 Malebogo Eluya

The views expressed in this work are solely those of the author.

For information contact: afiya.eluya@gmail.com

Interior and cover designed by Afroshapers.

ISBN: **978-1-312-58571-3**

Table of Contents

Dr Lebo

Preface

We all ought to eat healthy and nutritious diets, but unfortunately this isn't the case. Healthy eating is a privilege that many can't afford, and often those who can afford it still don't choose a healthy lifestyle. A nutritious diet is simply what our beautiful bodies demand to keep up with life. Everyone should understand this so well that a discussion is unnecessary, let alone a book about it. If we are willing to give our cars clean fuel and oil without compromise, then why not pay better attention to what we feed our bodies? Unfortunately, the reality is that we are not a healthy society and we are quite frankly eating our lives away. There are a number of factors influencing what we eat, how much we eat, and when we eat (if we are able to eat at all). *The Mindful Eater* is a simple and relatable discussion on modern-day attitudes towards food. This book teaches you how to pay greater attention to the moment-to-moment experience of eating, which will in turn help you improve your diet, manage food cravings, and lose weight. I have avoided scientific jargon so that absolutely anyone can use this to unlearn the bad and learn the good. I encourage mindful eating for our overall well-being. Imagine how many diseases could be avoided if we ate healthier! With its thought-provoking chapters, *The Mindful Eater* will surely change your life and (hopefully) the way you think about food and eating.

Introduction

My health is my wealth

I've been thinking about writing a book about mindful eating for some time. The inevitable moment when 'pen meets paper' couldn't be delayed any longer; there is an overwhelming need for informed, relatable discussions on all matters concerning diet and nutrition. I could have waited for traces of gray to creep into my hair before passing on this valuable knowledge to the next generation, but how could I have enjoyed the sunset years of my life and career if humanity was perishing right beside due to a lack of the knowledge that I am capable of sharing? Mindful eating has the power to save lives! Even if this book only impacts one life positively, I will be immensely satisfied, beloved reader! To see just one life lived longer, healthier, and happier would fill me with the great joy aligning with my calling and life purpose.

By the way, hello! I'm a dietician and nutritionist named Lebo, although I'm affectionately known as "Dr. Lebo" by my ever-growing troop of patients and followers. Please fetch yourself a glass of water and get comfortable because we are about to have a meaningful chat about your health and nutrition! The media has repeatedly hijacked the subject of eating in a bid to promote fad diets. This has been incredibly harmful for society, as many people have been steered towards eating habits that lead to obesity. Obesity and "weight loss" have become such focal issues that there is now a misconception emerging that if you are a person of normal weight then you are free to eat anything you want. I am here to change that narrative and will share some basic, life-saving truths. Through this book, I hope to positively influence your relationship with food and nutrition, regardless of your weight. Food can be an addictive 'drug' that can cause our early demise if mishandled.

Over the years of consulting as a dietitian, I have realized that a lot of people, even those living with a serious health condition (like diabetes), lack correct information when it comes to healthy eating. I have found that people are often confused by incorrect dietary information that they receive either from family members, the internet, and sometimes even from healthcare professionals. In recent times, however, I have been encouraged by the increasing number of people who are seeking out dietitians for dietary advice, rather than diving into the risky sea of diluted information that can be found on the internet.

When I first started private practice in 2015, most of my patients were referred to me by a doctor. Today, people are becoming more proactive about their well-being such that I am now seeing more patients who are self-referrals. Many of these patients are not sick but are interested in nutrition and lifestyle advice that can protect their health in the long run. It obviously excites me to know that people are starting to care more about the quality of their lives and their longevity. In fact, people are taking such an interest in their health, that our practice has a two month waiting list. I personally consult with between 20-30 clients a day (many of them self-referrals), which is a huge improvement from the 1-5 self-referrals we were seeing per day only a few years back.

I would like to think that this growth in nutritional awareness and self-referrals is in part influenced by my social media presence. I have been determined to leverage social platforms to educate the general public on nutrition in the name of a healthier, happier society. My social media accounts have generated a lot of interest locally, in Gaborone, as well as in neighboring South Africa, and even in Europe. The more I interact with people from different backgrounds, the more I realize how much misinformation there is about food on the internet... and how readily people will believe it. A classic example of such misinformation is that carbohydrates are fattening and make us gain weight. Another common misconception is that one has to eat fancy and expensive foods to be healthy.

What I thought people knew, in relation to what people actually know, has drastically changed the way I share health education with the public. While people seem to be becoming increasingly aware of the importance of regular physical activity, there still seems to be a knowledge gap where healthy eating is concerned. But I had to find a way on how to be able to get the general public to understand my message without being intimidating whatsoever. To increase the impact of my educational content, I avoid technical and scientific jargon as far as possible. I deliver my messages as simply and as relatably as I can, mainly in the local language of Setswana (even though I appreciate that not all my followers are from Botswana). My goal is to make information about healthy eating as accessible and understandable within my community as possible.

Having studied nutrition since secondary school in the 90s, I can tell you that nutrition (like any science) has evolved, and will continue to do so. Initially, the field's primary focus was on malnutrition and nutrient deficiencies; dietary guidelines were tailored to addressing these issues. Then the HIV/AIDS pandemic shifted focus to 'boosting the immune system' before antiretroviral therapies became available countrywide in the early 2000 (this was at least the case in Botswana and its surrounding region). During this time, extreme weight loss, known as "wasting syndrome" was a symptom associated with HIV/AIDS. While this is merely a personal theory without any scientific basis, I believe that the social stigma around HIV/AIDS, and therefore being thin, was a contributing factor to the obesity problem we currently face in our country. The downside for the slender was that even if they did suddenly gain weight, they were then perceived to be on ARVs and that the treatment was working well. Unfortunately, weight gain was celebrated as a sign of recovery. I believe that a lot of bad eating habits developed for people during this time. Instead of wasting syndrome, we now face an obesity pandemic.

In early 2020, Botswana (along with the rest of the world) was once again faced with a brutal pandemic: Covid 19. The world was brought to its knees by this invisible virus that held the power to completely shut down the world. I experienced the lockdown period as a scene from a horror movie. Every day we received news of people within our community who had died from the virus - both strangers and friends. Even the world's best scientists were at a loss of what to do. With restricted movements, even to the shops, many people developed 'hoarding' behaviors that included buying more food than needed. Again, I believe bad eating habits developed as a result.

In the days of lockdown, what else was one meant to do but entertain their stomach with food? Many of the clients that I am seeing today have experienced weight gain and other Noncommunicable Diseases (NCDs) as a result of the Covid period. Working from home, the emotional distress of losing loved ones, and the constant thrum of stress and fear all had a huge negative imperative on most people's health. What's more, lockdown and the threat of Covid 19 discouraged many people from attending their scheduled checkups and medical examinations. The gyms were empty and even opportunities to exercise outside were limited. Unfortunately, the government's efforts to combat Covid 19 meant that other public health threats, like NCDs, were neglected.

Today, COVID-19 may seem like a nightmare from the past, however, those of us who escaped this terrible virus are now faced with the longer-lasting threat of NCDs. I am beginning to see a lot of young patients (merely in their 20s and 30s) with conditions like hypertension and diabetes. Until recently, these conditions have been more common in older adults. Furthermore, morbid or extreme obesity is becoming increasingly common. It is not uncommon for me to consult with a young adult in their 30s weighing more than 120kg. As a practitioner, I find these trends extremely worrisome. It is for this reason that I am so passionate about public health efforts. I don't want to wait for a client to walk through once they are already suffering from a condition that needs to be managed; I want to help prevent the development of NCDs through education and information-sharing. As a company, Afiya Health and Dietetics Consultants (my practice), focuses on NCD prevention and screening activities. We often partner with the Ministry of Health's "Walk for Life", which is a governmental initiative intended to combat the rising NCD problem. I usually represent our company at these events by offering screening and professional information to the general public. At these events, people generally express a lot of interest in learning more about diet and nutrition. While most people still do not understand the role a dietitian can play in their health and wellbeing, I must say that there seems to be a very positive shift in awareness occurring due to our presence in the community.

This book is yet another tool through which I hope to share information and generate awareness around the importance of diet and nutrition. The chapters are carefully crafted and include personal stories and real-life testimonies intended to act as a wake-up call, as well as handy resources to assist a positive mindset-shift around nutrition and diet, especially in Africa. I hope that The Mindful Eater will have a generational impact because, at the end of the day, a healthy society is a happy society, and a happy society is a productive one. Our success and longevity depends upon good health: our future is only as bright as our eating habits. I am not only a dietitian, but a mother and a public servant burning with the desire to see a healthy society. Truthfully, I am just a *concerned citizen*. Without further ado, let's chat about a couple of topics, from healthy eating to practical dietary guidelines on a budget, and everything in-between.

Dr Lebo

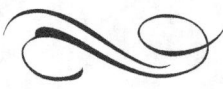

The Mindful Eater

Dr Lebo

Chapter 1

My Journey

I'd like to start by introducing myself and sharing a little of my story with you. My name is Lebo - or "Dr Lebo", as I'm affectionately known by my patients. However, I'd hate for you to take me for a mere academic, devoid of personality and life stories! So here's a bit about me: I grew up in the '70s and '80s, when one would dream of being either a nurse or a teacher. These two professions were undoubtedly symbolic of success and every family took pride in having a nurse or a teacher in the house. It never once crossed my mind that I would be called *Dr. Lebo one day… that* would have been way too far fetched! I wasn't one who concerned myself with dreaming high and far. I recall telling my parents that I planned to pursue typing when I finished form 3; this would mean dropping out of school. Dropping out wasn't a big deal to my mind. Neither of my parents graduated from university and yet we lived a comfortable life. At that age, I lacked motivation to work hard at school despite the fact that I was considered a very bright learner. In fairness, I was a 'lazy learner': just happy enough to pass and not at all interested in working hard enough to excel. The thing that I most enjoyed doing was drawing, even though I did not have much talent. What I lacked in talent, I certainly made up for in passion, however! I also took great joy in reading comic books and novels.

As it would happen, I became a mother at the age of seventeen, which inevitably interrupted my education. I was now nursing my beautiful child while trying to navigate my teenage life. The next three years were a wake-up call for me to take school and my education seriously. Even though I had tremendous family support, I literally had to grow up overnight. I consider myself extremely fortunate, in that I did not need to worry about fending for myself and my newborn child financially because my parents fully supported me. The turning point in our lives came when we abruptly decided to relocate to the United States in the 90s. Even though I did not know it at the time, this was to be a defining moment and a turning point in my life - especially with regards to my education and eventual career path.

The prospect of migrating to the land of infinite possibilities excited me and ignited my desire to further my studies. Upon arriving in the USA, I was admitted to the University of the District of Columbia, Washington DC. I was enrolled to study business administration. I worked odd jobs in order to take a couple of modules and earn a few credits each semester. However, my study plans shifted completely when I met a representative from another school, Howard University, at one of my school's career fairs. Howard University was offering a course I had never heard of before; the course was in "Nutritional Sciences". I had greatly enjoyed the topic of food and nutrition in Secondary School, so the course immediately grabbed my intention. I felt called to pursue it further.

Since I was attaining excellent grades for the program I was studying at that time, the Howard University representative admitted me If I could meet a few other requirements, then I would qualify to enroll in the more competitive Dietetics

5

program that accepted less than 30 students per year! Securing funding was going to be the tricky part as I was not actually in a financial position to attend such a prestigious university. I don't know how my father pulled it off, but after countless back-and-forth engagements, the Government of Botswana agreed to sponsor my studies. There I was, proudly attending classes at Howard University. Despite the usual ups-and-downs associated with academic life, I successfully graduated from Howard University in 2000.

A couple of months after completing my studies, I was on a plane back home to Botswana, leaving my family behind in Washington DC. My precious firstborn daughter was now under the full-time care of my mother. I cannot emphasize enough how much my parents' support carried me as far as I've come. Their constant love and care has shaped the person I am today. It was difficult arriving back in Botswana without them. For the first time ever I was literally on my own… and without a job! Nevertheless, I received an offer from the ministry of health within three months of my return. They were seeking a dietitian to join one of their HIV/AIDS programs. As this was my only offer, I willingly accepted, although I quickly discovered over the next nine months that working in a sickly hospital environment wasn't for me. Fortunately, I secured a permanent job with the Botswana Defence Force soon afterwards.

I largely accepted the position with the Botswana Defence Force because I was attracted to the unknown and the challenge it presented. Even though I was still working in a medical center, the culture and environment of the workplace was unusual... It was stress-free! I was content. In fact, I was happy showing up for work. Not a lot (beyond the bare minimum) was expected of me because, in the military, one works according to orders or instructions. During my time with the Defense Force, I also started neglecting my health and gaining weight. Yes, you heard me: I was a dietician who was being reckless with her diet and her health. I was predominantly working among men, which had led me to unintentionally adapt their eating habits - especially overeating. I was unaware that I was known as the 'fat dietitian'. But as I was young, I must say that it wouldn't have bothered me.

After a couple of years of the same daily routine, I ended becoming actively involved on the Defense Force's HIV/AIDS committee. My passion for public health deepened. I had the opportunity to present a lot of health education and, for the first time, I truly felt passionate about my work and sensed that it was more of a calling than a career. After some convincing, my employer agreed to sponsor my further studies in the United Kingdom. I attended another prestigious university, the University of Westminster, where I completed an MSc in Public Health Nutrition. A lot happened in my personal life after graduation that defined my career. I got married and fell pregnant with my second (and last) child all in the same year (2010). What should have been a very happy time in my life turned my world upside down! It proved to be one of the toughest seasons of my life.

Twenty-seven weeks into my pregnancy, something terrifyingly unexpected happened. I entered into premature labor and had to undergo an emergency delivery. I gave birth to a severely premature baby, weighing a little less than 1kg. After three months of ups-and-downs with my baby girl's health (which felt like decades), we were finally discharged from the hospital. I knew that my excess body weight was one of the contributing factors that led to my premature delivery. I had never really cared about my weight until that experience. I was a chubby child and then "the fat dietitian", so I knew how to let weight-related comments bounce off me. But nearly losing my daughter had been a rude awakening. Thankfully, my daughter came through this experience without any permanent health complications, but I needed to make some drastic changes regarding my health and weight.

I promised myself that I was going to enter my 40s in much better shape. I was still working for the Botswana Defense Force at this time, but my perspective shift prompted me to even leave my very comfortable job. After serving for the required period to pay off my sponsorship obligations, I re-entered academia to pursue my PhD at one of the local tertiary institutions. I derived immense benefits from being in an academic environment. There were many expectations to meet and stringent regulatory requirements to adhere to. The years I spent at the university were instrumental to my growth. It was, however, a stressful time too. While studying, I opened a private clinic with one of the local private hospitals. Hard work became the norm, and sleeping became a luxury!

I earned the title, 'Dr' and was earning a comfortable salary in academia, but the job was killing my spirit. I was losing myself! I had to make the very difficult decision to just walk away, even though I did not have a clear "Plan B". I quit my job during the height of the Covid 19 pandemic, but I trusted my strength and resolve. I focused on the only option I had at the time, which was my private clinic. Like most businesses, mine had zero clients (and therefore zero income) during the lockdown period. Nevertheless, I went to work every day during the lockdowns. The quiet period afforded me necessary time to reflect and ponder on the direction of my business. It was during this time that someone commented on my personal Facebook page (I wish I remembered his name now) that I should begin a Facebook page for my business. I took his advice without a script or a plan. Dr. Lebo arrived on social media in 2021, and my following grew steadily.

Stepping into the role of "Dr. Lebo" brought out exactly who I am as an individual. The real me: not as a wife, or a mom, or a professional, but as ME. Sometimes my colleagues thought I was being too personal, but I allowed my personality out. I liked sharing my experiences on my Facebook page. My odd mixture of both professional and personal messages seemed to motivate my readers. This is not to say that everyone was receptive to my messages; my following was not large at first. About a year later, however, my following blew up seemingly overnight. It has gotten to the point where I am somewhat of a public figure - it still shocks me! People constantly share feedback with me about how their lives have changed for the better since following my page, especially with regards to their health and nutritional knowledge. Since I have also struggled with obesity, sharing my story through social media has helped me work through my own challenges. My health is also benefiting because as I educate the public, I am joining in on the nutrition 'Challenges' I set for them. My current challenges are: "#MeatlessMonday"; "#GoGreen"; "#Brownies" and "#EverySipCounts" initiatives. Through these challenges, I encourage the public to make small positive changes to their diet. I share my personal story with you, beloved reader, in the hopes that you realize that I am not just an academic or a dietetics professional. I am a person just like you, who has had to overcome health challenges and learn to respect my body. We are in this together!

Here are some life lessons that I have learned:

1. Our lives are a reflection of the choices we make - both the good and the bad. This is true of our health too.

2. Certain changes are necessary in life. Don't be afraid to make them.

3. Your future demands that you make healthy decisions today, even if those decisions are tough!

4. Even if you do not see the results yet, keep going!

5. Your past mistakes provide you with an opportunity to learn from them and change your future. Don't waste them!

Chapter 2

The Time for Change

Fables should be taught as fables, myths as myths, and miracles as poetic fantasies. To teach superstitions as truths is a most terrible thing. The child mind accepts and believes them, and only through great pain and perhaps tragedy can he be in after years relieved of them. - **Hypatia of Alexandria**

We enjoy the incredible privilege of living in the most advanced era of technology and industrialization. Today's world and its advancements were barely imaginable ten years ago, let alone twenty or fifty years ago. The world is advancing at the speed of lightning in every field, including medical and health-related fields. Diagnostics, personalized medicine, and state-of-the-art technology are some of the drivers that have progressed the healthcare industry beyond our wildest dreams. "Progress" obviously offers enormous benefits, but it also comes with its fair share of challenges. Sometimes these challenges can actually take us ten steps backwards. For example, it is wonderful that everyone has access to a plethora of information these days, thanks to technology. Unfortunately, however, a lot of this information is incorrect, especially when it comes to health and diet. When the public are hooked on myths and notions that have no scientific basis, it makes the work of healthcare professionals very challenging indeed.

How does one go about busting myths that people have long-believed as the absolute truth? A professional should never criticize a patient's beliefs (even though it is tempting when one hears the absurd things that some have bought into). I have made a conscious decision that my approach will never be to blatantly discourage people who follow strange diets, but rather to let them experience the benefits of eating a diet scientifically proven to support their health. As people experience the health benefits of such a diet for themselves, their mindsets shift. This shift does not happen overnight; it takes time for people to trust you, even if you hold the credentials that I have. It is difficult, even for a professional, to compete with misinformation and dietary fads that promise miraculous results from drinking shakes and detox concoctions, or from eating slimming nuts.

Even without scientific evidence, I know that the public delights in testimonies and is willing to believe them blindly. People seldom seem to question the authenticity of such testimonies, especially if they are conveyed through social media. My mission was initially to nullify as much of the misinformation that is circulating as possible. I am well aware that it is a huge undertaking that sounds more like the sequel to James Bond's *Mission Impossible*. I soon realized that I was fighting a losing battle. It was not easy initially to admit defeat, but I had to gather my thoughts and think of another approach that would not paint me as a bitter health professional. I needed to be easily approachable and trustworthy before people would listen to the evidence-based information I had to offer.

Some people mistake my public visibility and social media influence as an overnight accomplishment that requires very little effort to maintain. The reality is that for the last two years or so, I have spent sleepless nights creating content for social media, as this is my tool for getting my professional voice out there to shift societal perceptions about diet and health towards factual, scientifically-based knowledge. When I first started posting messages about nutrition, I got a lot of backlash from people. Often their comments implied that I was "just afraid of the competition" and that I was criticizing products and treatments that were actually helping people. I came to realize that, to the public, healthcare professionals are notorious for criticizing 'alternative therapies'. I quickly became aware that I would have to be patient and put my personal feelings aside in the name of my mission. This said, I can't even begin to count the times that I have been tempted to just throw in the towel and give up!

I remember this one time that I made a post speaking out against some treatment that promoted quick weight loss by freezing body fat. I must admit that before I made the post I did not envisage the level of backlash I would receive on social media. Unfortunately, the person who had originally posted about doing this treatment was a well-known public personality.

The public assumed that I must be bitter against this person rather than that I truly believed that the treatment was a gimmick. After that post I thought the name of Dr. Lebo was in trouble. I was being painted as a bitter doctor who was jealous of another Motswana who was trying to make an honest living. I had to think fast because this was a make-or-break situation. There were some who were even demanding that I publicly apologize… even though my post did not mention any names!

In the end I decided to delete my post and made a new post in which I notified my audience of my intention to close my page. Wow, I received so many messages of support and encouragement in response. I was truly humbled to my core because it was so unexpected. I had been concentrating on the negative feedback of the minority (whose voices always seem loudest) and overlooking the people who were quietly supporting my work and experiencing genuine results. The influx of feedback that I almost instantly received entreating me not to close the page was certainly overwhelming. These strangers who had until now been dormant in my post comments suddenly sprang to life to offer support and to advocate for the continuation of the page. This told me that the information I was sharing was something they were hungry for. I also realized that many had been using my page as a way to verify information that was circulating in society.

I must admit that I receive many questions regarding fundamental truths: people want to differentiate between myths and facts. I don't want to simply answer these questions using my own feelings and opinions; I want to answer based on scientific truths that are widely accepted by scholars. Therefore, I need to read a lot and continually educate myself, especially when I am uncertain about a particular subject. As a professional, I have to ensure that the information I give out to the public is evidence based because I am well aware that I am always under the microscope, so to speak. Every piece of information that I share is not only dissected by the public but also by my peers, even though they may not always comment on my page. My greatest challenge has been mastering the art of being relatable to the public and delivering scientific information using simple language that anyone can understand without losing the message. The public is often bombarded with technical jargon that is meaningless to the ordinary citizen, and this technical information, in my opinion, frankly does not motivate behavioral change.

It is one thing to inform, but information is ineffective if people don't change their behavior. The fact that I have had personal experience struggling with weight and food (and that I am still a work in progress) has proved an advantage in regards to connecting with my clients and the public. Knowing that I have been down the same road as them makes me relatable. I can more easily understand what others are going through because I know what it is like from my personal experience. I have learned that sometimes professional experience is not enough on its own. Personal experience goes a long way both as a teacher and a testimony. To make a drastic health or lifestyle change, and then to sustain it, requires a complete mindset shift. The way we think and how we view ourselves can be a determining factor in how we live our lives. One who lacks a positive mindset is likely to fail because one critical comment from someone else can completely discourage you… especially comments from those who live around you. Many people have given up because they listen to the foundless opinions of other people. Other people become discouraged when the myths and gimmicks they believe in fail to bring about their desired results.

I have on occasion received comments that I am still fat, even though I was aware that I had lost some weight. Yes, these comments would make me feel miserable, but I always make an effort to talk encouragingly to myself and to remind myself of how far I have come. I know that I have made a lot of progress. And as for other people, I have learned not to expect compliments from them. Feedback is good, but sometimes it delays one's progress - especially when given without due consideration. On the whole, I think that most dietary advice has been provided very impersonally, using unrelatable technical jargon. When I read posts or articles on nutrition, I often find that it is either a cut-and-paste message (meaning that it had been used elsewhere in exactly the same manner), or the words used do not usually speak directly to the individual (meaning that it is impersonal).

I want to speak to the individual. This is one of the reasons why I decided to actively engage with social media, and it was also the motivation behind this very book. I know that there will be a number of people who will never read my messages, but I want to try a new approach with regards to re-educating the public on health and nutrition. As I prepare my messages, the question I always ask myself is: will people relate to this enough when they read it to make significant changes in their lives? I have, unsurprisingly, learned the most about how to effectively educate the public through my interactions with individual clients that I have consulted with at my clinic. Many of their statements are so similar to each other that it's almost as if I am responding to them by script. For example, many of them tend to share how difficult it is to be on a diet if the rest of the family is eating "normally". This is especially difficult for a woman who has to prepare two pots of food: one for herself and the rest for the family.

It is important to promote healthy eating within family units, however, one of the barriers to cultivating healthy eating habits is a limited, unadventurous diet where one repeatedly eats the same foods. I always remind my clients that the family shouldn't be forced to eat healthily. This said, the client should be committed to their dietary program and encourage family members to taste some of the healthy foods that they are eating, so as to dispel the myth that eating healthily means eating unappetizing food. Be patient with your family members until they are actually ready to make some dietary changes. The person who comes for a dietary consultation has a lot of influence on those around them and is able to spread the information they learn about healthy eating. When a client experiences positive results from following our program, they are especially likely to promote eating healthily and also to refer other people to the clinic for a dietary consultation.

When I first opened my clinic, I used to rely heavily on doctors' referrals to get clients through our doors. Over the past few years, however, new clients are increasingly being referred by satisfied existing clients. There is nothing so powerful as a personal testimony to encourage others to take a step in the direction of positive change too. Yes, people know about lifestyle-driven diseases, like diabetes and hypertension, but they often don't believe the message is directed at them. I understand that it is easy to believe that "it will never happen to me", either because of a lack of personal experience or out of fear. My intention is not to scare you, but I do want you to take lifestyle diseases seriously, because they can happen to you - or your mother, brother, friend, or another loved one. As a society, it is important to start making healthy changes to our diets. Many people can't face the idea of giving up certain foods, but my message is very clear: it is not about forbidding "bad" food but rather about learning to eat better for the benefit of one's overall health. Food can heal, but it can also cause disease.

Every day is a battle against the misinformation that people have read or have even been given by uninformed health professionals. For example, many people, including some of those living with diabetes, believe that brown sugar is healthier than white sugar. How has this myth survived? And after so many years, how do I begin to unravel this misinformation and dispel these kinds of myths? With this being said, no food is "bad" in itself; it depends on how it is eaten. To explain, consider someone who has a habit of drinking several cups of tea per day, with four teaspoons of brown sugar in each cup. In this scenario, sugar definitely becomes a health hazard. On the other hand, sugar is not a health hazard for someone who drinks tea infrequently with just a little white sugar. As a society, we have a long way to go to combat misinformation and become healthy, but I am confident that we will get there. I hope that this book will enable reliable dietary information to reach a larger portion of the population.

Here are some tips on engaging with diet & health information:

1. When seeking reliable Information, turn to peer-reviewed and articles published in reputable journals. Be skeptical of information published on unverified websites.

2. Reputable websites include those of government departments like the Ministry of Health, or those of international organizations like the World Health Organization.

3. Just because many people are doing something doesn't mean that it is a good idea.

4. It's always a good idea to have a one-on-one consultation with a reputable dietician who has knowledge of your health conditions.

5. Following a personalized diet (tailored to your health conditions) is better than following generalized dietary advice.

6. Healthcare is a regulated profession. In Botswana, healthcare professionals are regulated by the Botswana Health Professions Council. If you are unsure of someone's credentials, contact the regulatory bodies to double-check.

Dr Lebo

Chapter 3

Reality check

It is very different attending to very sick patients in hospital compared to consulting with the 'healthy' who come to me as outpatients. Most of the patients who I consult with in my clinic come in for weight loss. Usually, these patients assume that weight is their only issue. However, obesity is considered a disease, so I often insist that these clients do other basic tests for conditions such as hypertension, diabetes, and sometimes even thyroid issues. Unsurprisingly, there is almost always a test result that shocks the client, as they assumed they were "healthy" despite their weight. Other times, I suggest tests to dispute a self-diagnosed condition that a client incorrectly assumes is related to their struggle with weight.

When I talk with people, I usually find that they are in denial about the extent that their weight negatively impacts their health. Some believe their body pains and elevated blood pressure is due to some factor other than their weight. The truth is, excess body weight and excessive weight gain are a common cause of these symptoms. Some people get to the point where they have a health scare or have to start medical treatment before they finally admit to themselves that dietary changes are necessary. I often tell my patients that doctors prescribe medication as a last resort when they lack trust in the patient to take good care of themself and their health. The doctor would probably have told their patient to make some lifestyle changes in the earlier stages of a disease's onset, but then the patient comes back either in the same or a worse condition, forcing the doctor to aggressively medicate their condition. Even then, the patient may say the doctor was too quick to medicate, even though they were probably given enough time and guidance to safely treat their condition by making lifestyle changes.

With all this said, it is usually the patient who is experiencing a compromised quality of life who is eager to make lifestyle changes, rather than those forced by a medical scare. For example, a patient who can't walk long distances, or who has trouble sleeping due to excess body weight is more likely to want to make lifestyle and dietary changes. During counseling, their dietician will know that it is critical to address issues that are affecting quality of life in order for the patient to address the root of the problem. Excess weight can affect many aspects of people's lives; one may not have enough energy to play with their kids or be prevented from having a healthy intimate relationship with their partner. The counseling session is a key to helping a patient understand what their lives could be. The dietician will ideally be able to inspire eagerness for positive change. Without scaring the patient, it is also the dietician's responsibility to make the client aware of the health implications that will result if changes are not made. After talking about the scary stuff, I try to bring out the positives once more by reminding the client that they are always in control of their own health journey (rather than us healthcare professionals). Positive change may start off with something simple like starting a medical diary to keep track of their blood pressure, blood sugar, and medications. Accurate medical records go a long way in helping a healthcare professional to help you. Some patients try to recall their medical history off the top of their heads, but it is unrealistic to correctly recall every detail, including medication names and dosages.

As a healthcare practitioner, it is important not to only focus on food but also on tools that will empower and encourage the patient. It is usually after learning such tools that the patient starts to get excited about this new way of living that puts them in control of their health while getting their weight under control. A patient that feels helpless is more likely to feel overwhelmed and give up prematurely. Sadly, I have witnessed patients giving up before experiencing the benefits to our programmes. I must admit that this breaks my heart, not because I am losing a client, but because I know their quality of life will continue to deteriorate due to poor health caused by their diet and malnutrition. As such, my approach today tends to focus on achieving short-term successes that systematically boost the confidence and commitment of both my motivated and unmotivated clients alike. To explain, I have found that even a patient who is making good progress becomes discouraged when they focus on how far they still have to go. However, when they rather focus on how far they have already come 'now,' they feel proud of their achievement. My precious reader, I celebrate you if you have already started to address your health, and if you haven't, I encourage you to start today! As you read this book, remember to focus on your wins and keep going.

I usually discourage anyone from making dietary changes in their life from a place of focusing on the challenges. I urge them to instead set their eyes and their goals, and the rewards that will result from achieving those goals. Often the prospects of feeling lighter, looking good, and gaining energy motivate us despite the challenges. For most people, self-control with regards to what to eat and when to eat is a far greater challenge than feeling hungry when implementing dietary changes. Hunger itself is often more psychological than physical. I often illustrate this to clients by pointing out that they can easily go the whole day (or most of the day) without even remembering to eat if they have a hectic schedule. With this being said, forgetting to eat for an entire day is also not healthy. A hectic schedule can also impact the time one realistically has to prepare and eat healthy meals. For this reason, it is critical that companies and organizations begin considering nutrition and health as a crucial part of their employee's health and wellbeing.

Truth be told, the majority of people spend most of their time in the workplace, rather than at home. We must begin questioning whether these work environments are enabling good eating habits, or whether they are exacerbating poor habits. In my opinion, most organizations do not consider nutrition and health to be a priority (judging by the lack of policies to promote health in the workplace). In all seriousness, it is in a company's best interests to promote their employees' health, as this would reduce human capital problems, like absenteeism and low productivity, which are likely caused by lifestyle and health factors. Simple acts like providing healthy meal choices in the cafeteria and thinking twice before serving unhealthy foods at company meetings can make a huge difference. I am always shocked when I realize that certain company cultures have normalized unhealthy habits, such as tea times where almost all employees sit down to drink sugary beverages and eat greasy foods, like fat cakes and hot chips (or fresh chips as we call them in Botswana). While these habits may feel like harmless pleasures, they are in fact deadly. How can a company expect their employees to perform to their full potential if their eating habits are suboptimal? Consider too the impact on entire family units if the breadwinner develops a chronic illness. On a larger scale, the health system becomes burdened as the number of people requiring care and treatment for chronic health conditions grows. It is, therefore, in the best interest of society as a whole to adopt a multi-sectoral approach to health, nutrition, and wellness.

I am obliged by my passion for public health and wellbeing to remind us all of a few truths that might have conveniently been overlooked within all spheres of our ailing society. One of these truths is that an unhealthy society negatively impacts the productivity and growth of our society as a whole. The strain that is being placed on the health system by a largely unhealthy population entirely is avoidable. We surely do not need science to tell us (though science does tell us) that there is a direct correlation between the health of people and their productivity. Again, a correlation exists between employee productivity and the success of an organization. If companies better prioritized the health of their people, in the same way that they strive to create safe physical working environments, many absenteeism due to sickness could be avoided.

Please take note that when I speak about an unhealthy society, that discussion is relevant to both you and me. We are a part of that society, and the reality is that if either you or I get sick because we are eating poorly, our lifestyle illnesses will have an impact on our families, our colleagues, and the wellbeing of our society as a whole. Take a moment to consider how many people, especially in your immediate family, would be affected if your health declined. With this in mind, next consider if you are satisfied with your health and your eating habits? How much money do you spend on foods that your body does not necessarily need? Are you aware that overindulgence in food invariably ends in tears of regret down the road? And one final question: what are you waiting for before you start taking good care of your health and eating habits?... A heart attack? Hypertension? Diabetes? Surprisingly, we often take greater care over how we fuel our cars than how we fuel our bodies. No one would pour dishwashing liquid or cooking oil into their car's fuel tank as they recognize that this would do damage to the car's ability to run long-term. We know a car needs petrol or diesel, and so that is what we give it. However, we don't think twice about what we feed our bodies; we end up consuming all sorts of harmful foods that impact our long-term wellbeing. Your body is your greatest asset, so be sure you are treating it with even greater care than you would devote to your most prized material possession.

I realize that this chapter may have been a little hard to digest, but I strongly believe that we need to take a good look at ourselves. We need to be brave enough to ask ourselves the hard questions and to stop hiding reality before it's too late. After all, a healthy mother, a healthy father, and healthy kids is a recipe for a happy home and a healthy nation. I'm sure you're starting to get the picture! While this message may be overwhelming, remember that you hold the power to turn your health and future around. The important thing is to make the necessary lifestyle changes as soon as you can to prevent long-term health complications. I urge you to choose health today!!

Dr Lebo

Chapter 4

Dealing with cravings

We have been brainwashed into craving a diet that is killing us. What we believe tastes good is generally what we have been socially conditioned to enjoy. - **Jane Velez-Mitchell**

I have worked as a healthcare professional in both the public and private sector. During my years of service, I have come to realize that people will always offer an excuse for their poor health and the diet they eat. People seem to be entirely unwilling to own up and take responsibility for their poor lifestyle choices when it comes to their diet and health. If we are not careful, the excuses we make for eating poorly will catch up with us and prevent us from living healthy, purposeful lives. One of the chief excuses clients give me for their poor eating

37

habits (and I have heard this over and over again) is having cravings. Yes everyone blames it on cravings!

Well, what are cravings? Most of us have experienced an intense urge to eat certain foods. More often than not, these foods tend to be sugary, salty, or fatty (or all three!). You may feel increasingly excited as you imagine how it will taste and how you'll feel eating it. The truth is that cravings do happen once in a while, and this urge usually goes away if resisted. Nowadays, however, people increasingly give in and satisfy their cravings, to the point that an addiction is developed. Think about it: when a person experiences an intense urge to drink a fizzy drink or an energy drink almost daily, is this just an innocent craving or has it reached the point of addiction? I believe you know the answer to this. There are certain habits and addictions that we tend to justify as being better than others. I always laugh when I hear people saying that their 'only' weakness is sugary foods because they don't even drink alcohol… as if to justify one bad habit over another! Avoiding alcohol does not justify eating excess sugar. It's like stealing from a supermarket but saying you're innocent because you drive under the speed limit.

As a dietitian, I see hundreds of clients per week. I have noticed that whenever people fail to adhere to a certain diet or healthy lifestyle, it is always linked to both good and bad eating habits. It is unusual for a person to have only good or only bad habits. Both types of habits usually exist side by side. For example, someone can be very strict about eating what is considered a healthy diet during the week, but then they relapse and overindulge in alcohol and junk food over the weekend. Perfection is not part of human nature, so I always encourage people not to feel too bad when their bad habits get the best of them. However, I also encourage them not to get too comfortable with these bad habits. I do not, however, want to lecture you in this book. Rather, my intention is to provide every reader with a life-changing tool to support their health (because our health is truly our wealth). As such, I have put together some tips on how to overcome challenging bad habits.

10 ways to overcome bad eating habits:

1. **The first step is to acknowledge what your weaknesses are when it comes to food**. Do you overindulge in sugar or another particular food? Do you fantasize about it to the extent that you cannot seem to

go a day without eating it? When one admits that a dietary habit is a problem, it is then easy to overcome it by coming up with specific, goal-driven solutions. For example, instead of having three teaspoons of sugar in your tea, you might reduce it to two.

2. **Avoid triggers that feed your bad habits**. Some people develop certain eating habits based on the habits of the people they spend time with. These habits could be formed with people in the workplace, at school, or in social gatherings. Some people eat fat cakes at work, for example, because it is the culture of that particular workplace: everyone eats fat cakes for breakfast. Keeping busy during tea time or lunchtime can distract one from being influenced and yielding to peer pressure. One can read a book or take a power nap to avoid eating unnecessarily.

3. **Having a written plan is very helpful.** It is easier to commit to something that has been written down. Just as having a shopping list helps one to stick to the plan, so too does writing out your intentions. Creating a meal plan for the week helps one to avoid bad habits and

incorporate good ones. Meal plans are also good for the pocket because one has a clear shopping list, which also helps avoid compulsive buying and eating.

4. **Eat home-cooked food more frequently.** Preparing meals at home, especially during the week, helps one to avoid buying poor quality foods that are often more expensive too. Preparing food to take to work with you will also help prevent compulsive eating. Even if you cannot do this every day, try to commit to at least three days where you eat home-prepared meals at work.

5. **Drink water.** This is so simple that it possibly sounds cliche, but drinking water can curb cravings for sugary beverages significantly (especially when the weather is hot).

6. **Avoid foods and beverages that feed another bad habit.** For example, some people love coffee and tea (substances that are not necessarily a health concern in themselves), but their consumption of these substances increases their sugar intake. Over time, they may develop a sugar addiction. While they may think they crave

coffee or tea, their body is actually using these cravings as an excuse to take in more sugar.

7. **Avoid eating while doing other activities**. It is not a good idea to watch tv while chewing on a snack. Mindless eating can easily result in overeating.

8. Avoid **shopping when hungry as this may activate cravings**. It is advisable to eat at home before going to the shops, even if you are simply going to the mall to spend time recreationally. The habit of eating before going into shopping spaces helps avoid mindless eating.

9. **Eating at home before attending a social event**. Eating at home before going to a social event, such as a wedding, minimizes the likelihood of overindulgence and unnecessary eating. The same advice applies to the working class and schoolgoers. Eat at home to avoid the temptation of eating unhealthy foods while out.

10. **Take care of your mental health.** Keep your mental health status in check by seeking necessary help when you are feeling stressed. This healthy habit will help you manage stress-related eating. Other activities that keep

the mind occupied, such as talking to a friend when feeling overwhelmed, can also help manage stress.

Final advise: no more restrictions

I focus on mindful eating with my clients. This is a non-judgmental awareness of the physical and emotional sensations associated with eating. To be clear, mindful eating is a way of eating, not a diet per se. In other words, mindful eating is all about being aware of how we feel when we eat. Given that most clients I consult with have tried all sorts of restrictive diets or exercise regimes with little success, I now start by giving them a simple rule: IF IT IS NOT WRITTEN, IT HASN'T BEEN DONE. This basically means that without a self-written and self-directed meal plan (created under the guidance of a dietitian), it is not doable. It is very easy for one to think that they are eating well based on their own ideas about food, in conjunction with faulty recollections about what has truthfully been eaten. For example, it is human nature to recall only the healthy foods eaten and conveniently forget the unhealthy snacks eaten between meals, sometimes totally unconsciously.

My approach avoids radical cleanses and does not eliminate certain foods. I do not advocate for clearing out your cupboards, nor do I suggest fads and quick fixes. I believe that mindful eating is an effective approach that guides more mindful food choices, potentially leading to weight loss and healthier eating overall. Eating mindfully is not about feeling guilty or regretful about certain foods you eat, but rather about being intentional and mindful with eating. Mindful eating involves being present while cooking or eating; it involves slowing down to truly savor our food without any judgment, guilt or anxiety. This approach encourages you to spend less time focusing on your weight and the storylines around it. By embracing mindful eating, people naturally tend to find the weight that is right for them.

Mindfulness asks us to take a kinder, gentler approach to eating. The focus is not necessarily on changing the food we eat (though it can be); it's about changing our thinking towards food. For example, rather than thinking about how some foods are fattening, focus your attention on learning how to better prepare food, the right portions to take, and learning to take pleasure from really tasting the food on your plate (instead of overindulging). Mindful eating is rooted in thoughtfulness and choice analysis. Part of mindful eating is to consider the "why" of eating. Ask yourself: what is my intention for eating? Are you starving or do you just eat because food is available and you can afford it? Are you eating to satisfy a craving, or because it is what your body needs nutritionally?

One of the greatest benefits of practicing mindful eating is that we actually enjoy our food more, but in smaller portions. If you have a negative attitude, or if you feel deprived, you are very likely to fail. For this reason, I cannot underestimate the benefit of physical consultation with a dietician or even attending virtual support groups. Virtual support groups are for helping one adjust their mindset and for holding you accountable on your mindful eating journey. Nobody better understands what you're going through than others that are in the same situation. The combination of expert and peer support is invaluable. It can feel overwhelming to implement mindful eating practices by yourself. Food is everywhere and everybody is trying to get us to eat more! Having a support team cheering you on can make all the difference, especially if you have someone who is both knowledgeable and objective, like a dietitian, guiding your steps.

Below are a few tips on how to follow Mindful eating:

1. Avoid the notion of dieting; rather talk about mindful eating.

2. Don't bend to cravings: eat because you are hungry.

3. Make peace with food.

4. Don't eat without a plan.

5. Listen to your stomach when it says, "I am full" and learn how your body feels when you have overindulged.

6. Food is not a remedy for your feelings. Do not use sadness, happiness, boredom, or anger as an excuse to eat.

7. Respect your body enough to listen to it.

8. Learn to say "no" without feeling guilty. In our culture it is considered rude to refuse food when offered, but your body and your health is yours to protect.

9. Be confident in your decisions regarding food, especially when your body is rejecting a particular food.

10. Lastly, know that healthy food does not mean healthy habits. One can gain weight by inappropriately eating healthy foods.

One should also ask themselves these key questions:

1. **Why?** Why do you eat? Is it because it is the normal time to eat, or has something triggered you to eat? For example, did you see someone else eating and all of a sudden feel hungry?

2. **When?** When do you want to eat? Is it based on feeling hungry or simply because it is lunchtime and everyone expects you to eat at that time?

3. **What?** What do you want to eat? How do you allocate money to food? Do you work your budget around what you are going to eat or do you buy according to your budget? Focus on what is nutritionally adequate rather than what you can afford.

4. **How?** How do you eat? Are you sacrificing your nutritional requirements because, for example, your budget can only afford two chicken pieces (not enough protein)? Are you willing to sacrifice the chicken and rather buy a cheaper plant-based protein source that will allow you to fully meet your nutritional protein requirement?

5. **How Much?** How much do you eat? Do you base your portions on what you dish out or rather on the type and the number of ingredients you use during cooking?

A final word of advice for this chapter: don't ever feel pressure to eat a certain way or to certain portion sizes just because you are from a certain tribe or of a certain age and gender. I am often told by clients that I should understand and excuse their poor eating because they are from a certain region known for its meat-eating habits, even if that person is no longer staying there.

Chapter 5

Stories of Hope

Nothing is as powerful as hearing true stories and testimonies. We all love a happy ending and often it is upon learning about other people's success stories that we find the motivation to pursue our journeys to victories. Similarly, your testimony of health and dietary transformation could one day motivate others to change their lifestyles for the better. Witnessing someone losing weight and becoming a normal weight after being obese is more powerful than a speech on the importance of losing weight. Over the years, I have had the extreme privilege of witnessing countless transformations and seeing lives change before my eyes. These success stories have been extremely encouraging for me personally as I continue serving as a dietitian and nutritionist in Botswana.

When I started running my clinic back in 2015, I longed to share the positive outcomes and happy endings witnessed in the clinic with the public. This desire was not driven by the need to market my practice, but from a place deep within me that longs to see other people encouraged by the true stories of ordinary citizens so that they too might begin choosing a lifestyle and dietary habits that can improve their overall health and effectively manage any existing conditions. Due to the strict code of ethics on patient confidentiality, I obviously could not, and still cannot share much. I worry that someone who has a certain disease may not seek help if they are feeling hopeless about their situation, but that their hope can often be restored if they hear stories of other people who have successfully overcome similar challenges. Oftentimes, people's negative opinions are not necessarily true, especially when it comes to remedial options for their conditions. A personal testimony goes a long way towards challenging misguided opinions.

I remain eternally grateful for social media platforms, like Facebook, because the people engaging on those platforms are often willing to share their positive feedback and testimonials freely and publicly, even if they are not necessarily my direct clients. When I first became active on social media in 2020, I lacked a clear direction of how I wanted to deliver my message to the public. I knew that I didn't want to be too formal or too intimidating, however. At times I posted on issues unrelated to health or nutrition, but my intention was to build a profile as "Dr. Lebo": someone knowledgeable who is also human and approachable. I wanted my followers to feel welcome to ask questions and to comment freely when I do discuss serious issues, without feeling ashamed. I wanted to create a safe space for everyone to learn about health and diet, regardless of their educational background or socio-economic status. Just two years, I think that is exactly what Dr. Lebo's social media platform has become.

One cannot control other people's opinions on social media, and these can sometimes be quite nasty and negative. I have had some unpleasant experiences where I have felt personally attacked but, fortunately, the majority of my followers are very supportive. I am overwhelmed by the way that they always seem to come to my defense when disparaging comments arise.

The positive testimonials I receive on social media draw many people to the clinic for a personal consultation. Of the great number of clients who I have seen over the years, there are a few who have had a particularly powerful impact on my professional life. I think you will benefit from hearing these stories, and I share them within the bounds of confidentiality and without violating any doctor-client privilege.

The first testimony I wish to share is that of an elderly gentleman, somewhere in his 70s, who came to the clinic recently. He had a history of diabetes and was already on medication to manage it. With elderly clients, mindset is usually the greatest challenge to overcome. If they have been told something else at any time, and never been given an alternative option by previous doctors, they are often unwilling to change their minds. For this reason, gaining the patient's trust is very important. My professional judgment told me that, with guidance and diet therapy, this patient could manage his diabetes without medication. He surprised me by being very open to learning, which lays the foundation for every success story. Nevertheless, I knew that I had to be careful not to overwhelm him while at the same time empowering him to take control of his condition. After thoroughly educating him on how to self-monitor blood sugar levels at home, I taught him how his food intake affects his blood sugar reading, and provided him with proof thereof. One thing that diabetes patients are very familiar with is severe food restrictions and the countless "dos" and "don'ts". With self-monitoring techniques, however, this patient was able to regain his freedom. He quickly began to realize that certain foods or portion sizes affected his blood sugar levels, and he was able to self-correct without the doctor adjusting his medications. What is most memorable about this gentleman, however, is that his doctor ultimately took him off the diabetes medications that he thought he was going to be taking for the rest of his life.

Age certainly does not mean that a patient is without hope. Because this gentleman was motivated to achieve better health, his journey was made much easier and his rewards were greater. His testimony humbled me and I felt a great sense of achievement with this particular client. I'd like to share some other motivational stories with you, my precious reader, because we often think that changing our diet is "mission impossible". This is because most diets out there are so restrictive that it almost feels like one is not allowed to eat at all. This is not our approach. At our clinic, we don't allow clients to go hungry, and we pride ourselves in ensuring that our clients are supported and truly believe in their own capabilities to succeed. While we provide our clients with the necessary support, it is unfortunate that a health transformation journey can often be a very lonely journey, taken solo.

Initially, I used to allow clients to be accompanied to their consultations by someone of their choosing for the purpose of support. During one such accompanied consultation, I met with two ladies who ended up both wanting to enroll in our weight loss program. I could tell they were using each other as a "security blanket", so my gut instinct was that they both lacked the resolve to truly succeed at the program. Against my better judgment, I enrolled them both. As expected, one of the ladies eventually dropped out, but (to my surprise) the other remained. I had warned her that she may feel like dropping out, but she felt confident enough to carry on with the program alone. A year later her weight had reduced from 127 kg to 95 kg.

Even though I no longer see this client frequently, I follow her journey closely on social media and her progress never ceases to encourage and inspire me. This student has now become a teacher! When I post the progress reports of my anonymous clients, most people do not get to hear the full story behind that journey. One of the amazing things this lady has done is to share her journey publicly, with great honesty and transparency regarding both the good things and the challenges. One of the unspoken truths about weight loss is that it often comes with a toxic habit of directing negative comments towards yourself. Some people who struggle with obesity gain back the weight because they develop an idea that they looked better when overweight, or because they fear that other people will suspect that their weight loss is due to illness. Societal pressures and the thoughts of others pose a challenge to the weightloss journey.

Just as it is physically noticeable when someone gains, for example, 20kg, so too will it be noticeable when one loses 20kg. The feedback from those around you regarding your physical changes may not always be positive… in fact it can be quite demoralizing! At our clinic, we psychologically prepare our clients for such feedback, which is another reason why our programmes are so effective. I have had a lot of clients whose partners cannot cope with the client's drastic physical changes because they feel threatened by the increased self-confidence that accompanies their transformation. When someone looks better, they tend to feel better about themselves too. The resultant change in their behavior can be overwhelming for those closest to them. While navigating these interpersonal dynamics, it is important to remember that transformation is about being healthier, not just about changing the physical appearance.

When I first started the clinic, our clients were mainly women. Over the years, however, we have seen a significant increase in the number of men who are interested in improving their health through diet therapy, and this trend is encouraging indeed! As a professional, I have come to understand the unique dietary needs of men. Ultimately, one of my long-term plans is to open a clinic that focuses specifically on men's health. I enjoy helping men regain control of their health without being pushed or pressured. One of the reasons why men shy away from seeking help is because they are often made to feel disempowered when it comes to making health-related decisions. If I had but one wish, it would be for all people to believe in their own capability to change their health, and to avoid depending too heavily on the many mixed and confusing messages circulating in the media and society.

Dr Lebo

Chapter 6

#Pay

There is a great illusion that we have tolerated from one generation to another, and this is the notion that the world, country, or other people owes us something. We seem to believe that if we remain seated and wait long enough, we will magically receive everything we wish for. Unfortunately, we continue to raise entitled generations of people who truly believe that the best of life comes for free. I mean, let's admit it, we have all wished to wake up one day with a million dollars in our bank accounts, or to become a great success, but at some point most of us have to realize that life simply does not work that way. There is a price attached to everything we want (and even need). I religiously use this hashtag on my social media and various communications: #PAY. I use this hashtag to debug the notion that the journey to health and lifestyle transformation is a free one.

The life we dream of comes at a price: the car we want to drive has a price tag, the family we want has a price to it too, as does every other element that makes up the lifestyles and bodies we dream of and envy. Whatever you desire to have will remain a mere wish unless you are willing to #PAY. Sadly, we are so conditioned to expect handouts and giveaways that the idea of paying a price scares us. In fact, we are so fixated on success and "end products", that we are blind to the journey that is required to get us there. We need to understand that there is a price to be paid to get over the finish line. Don't fall into the trap of focusing on the transformed person without acknowledging what they have really gone through to achieve drastic weight loss and lifestyle transformation.

We have been made to believe that there is a 'magic pill' that melts away excess body weight in the blink of an eye. There are a lot of products on the market that give the impression that someone can eat whatever they want and still lose weight without any exercise. It has been proven that these products are completely ineffective in the long run. One of my biggest frustrations is trying to convince people that shortcuts are not sustainable. People spend a lot of money trying these products that promise miraculous weight loss only to experience no real results. However, any weight loss that is achieved using these products is generally regained in excess the moment the person stops using the product. Weight loss is actually less of an issue than long-term weight management. We need to focus on being mindful of what we eat and what our bodies need.

If you try to take the shortcut to weight loss, you are likely not to learn the lifestyle habits (like self-control, and discipline) required to maintain a lower weight. In my years practicing as a dietitian, I have seen many clients who seem highly motivated during their initial consultation but who, unfortunately, end up not being able to cope in the program. Sometimes this surprises me, but I have also come to realize that some clients want to say the "right things" in a consultation - be it to convince me, or to convince themselves, that they are serious about our transformation program. These clients do not understand that transformation is not just about weight loss but about completely changing how one views food and one's relationship to it. After completing the programme, one shouldn't go back to previous eating habits that will cause the excess weight to return.

In my opinion, clients who enroll in the program without any expectations about what it involves are usually the most successful. Perhaps the reason for this is that they are willing to listen to advice and learn about the programme without questioning the process too much. Questions are fine in and of themself, but when people believe the false dietary information that is circulating out there and use questioning as a way to try and "catch their dietitian out", then they are stacking the odds of success against themselves. Please remember that dieticians are trained professionals who have received their information and training from reliable sources. You can trust their guidance.

Even when clients come in for a consultation without clear expectations, they generally do tend to think that our programmes will include many dietary restrictions, due to their previous experiences of "dieting". I am always upfront with my clients that there will be good and bad days. Even when one is not on a diet, there will be times of heightened cravings, and other times of more discipline. The idea is to get through the tougher days without giving in or getting caught up in unhealthy habits again. Because most people are conditioned to expect quick fixes, I am often asked by people during their first consultation how much they will be spending as if they are buying something from the shop shelf and expecting to walk away in an instant.

I compare the experience of following a transformation programme with that of going to school. Its value is not truly appreciated until after one has graduated. What one needs to do is focus on the learning journey until they get there. If one focuses on mastering the tools and implementing the knowledge during their transformation programme, one can ultimately become their own dietitian. I have personally taken that journey (as an individual, not as a dietician). I know from first-hand experience that it is not easy but that it is definitely worth the effort and investment. Imagine attending workshops and social events where there are lots of tempting foods and having to have the self-control to avoid overindulging.

I do not want to make it sound like I have had stellar self-control at all times, but I have learned how to become a mindful eater. It is important to listen to our bodies because they send out some signals while we are eating that let us know if our bodies actually agree with our food choices. For example, bloating is a warning signal that you are exceeding your body's capacity to process the food consumed. Some signs we attribute to something else other than food. Another example is changes in the skin, which is the first organ to express when one is not eating right. Some people may experience a change in their complexion or pimple breakouts. These are ways that our bodies give us feedback about the food we are feeding it.

Our food habits are most tested when we are in unfamiliar environments, especially while traveling or eating out. How does one avoid temptation and order what should be eaten? This can become especially challenging if someone else is paying for your meals, such as an employer. Discipline is most crucial when it is difficult to exercise. Try to stick to your normal routine even when in a different environment. To elaborate: if you do not eat meat on Mondays when at home, then avoid eating meat on Mondays no matter where you are. Discipline is a currency that you use to #Pay for the results you want to see.

Expecting perfection is unrealistic, but try to stay focused on the goal post despite the challenge. It is important to be kind to yourself if you mess up from time to time, but do not allow yourself to become so comfortable that you end up stuck in bad eating habits. It takes a lot of mental strength because transforming one's health is a solo journey, even if you have a supportive family. Sometimes our loved ones actually encourage our bad eating habits unintentionally. It may be something as small as offering you food that you have a weakness for, or simply eating that food around you. How does one resist? The problem is that if you give in, you may be flooded with feelings of guilt or loss of control. To fight this battle, it is important to have a good relationship with food (avoid attaching negativity to food). All people struggle with the restricted freedom of eating whatever they want, anytime and in unrestricted quantities.

In some cases feeling hungry or having cravings isn't the issue. Rather, it's a lack of control over one's diet. Whenever a client tells me that they have some kind of physical side effect while on a weight loss program, I ask them if they tend to spend the whole day without eating, either due to a tight work schedule or because of forgetting to eat. The answer is almost always yes. I then explain to them that our minds often play tricks on us to make us believe that when the body is denied food or fed in small portions, we get sick. I don't encourage starvation as a weight loss method, but it is important to distinguish between real physical hunger and psychological hunger.

Commitment is another key currency used to purchase the body and life that you desire. Commitment can be a difficult currency to #pay in, because in addition to the actual financial implications, one has to be willing to deal with the emotional rollercoaster of feelings that goes along with unlearning bad habits and learning new ones. On this note, one must be aware that there is a financial cost to enrolling in a transformation program too. This is not simply a once-off payment. The greater your weight loss goals, the longer you will be required to commit to the program, and thus the higher the price. Even if you have medical insurance, it is important that you are prepared to cover the full financial amount, should your medical coverage be exhausted.

Remaining unhealthy should not be optional because, in the long run, the costs of poor health will be higher than pursuing health habits now and may even cost one one's life. At the end of all the hard work, it is truly worth it. Most of our clients celebrate their improved quality of life as the weight just keeps coming off! What initially seems like a small achievement results in big lifestyle gains, such as one being able to tie their shoe laces or having improved energy, confidence and intimacy with their partner. Even after many years and many success stories, I am always most awed by the change in a client's self-confidence through a transformation programme. Sometimes the change is noticeable as early as the end of the first week, when they come in for a follow-up consultation full of excitement for 'surviving' the first week's struggles. All I can say is that if a client is patient and willing to go through the ups and downs... their end result will be rewarding.

All the success stories shared in this chapter (as well as those that I have not shared) came at a high price. These clients paid with the following:

❖ Discipline

Motivation may get you through my door for an initial consultation, but only discipline will ensure that you get through my program, having claimed your health, your life and your happiness back in the process.

❖ Finances

There is a financial cost attached to consulting a dietician, as well as a cost attached to the food and meal plans that ensure you are eating what is right and healthy.

❖ Time

You need to make time to make the necessary changes that will support your desired outcomes. Dedicate your time to pursuing the health transformation you need.

Conversely, the unfortunate stories of people who have not succeeded in changing their diet and health in time have also paid a heavy price with regards to the following;

❖ Health

If you do not take care of your health today, you will end up paying the price with unavoidable chronic illness or even death.

❖ Happiness

It is difficult to truly enjoy your life when you are overweight, especially when your weight leads to sickness or limits your activity.

❖ Finances

If you do not invest in eating right today, you will eventually pay for your bad eating habits in the form of medical bills directly resulting from illness associated with your long-term eating habits.

❖ Career

Poor eating habits can affect your health in ways which can lead to poor performance at work, and possibly resulting in the loss of your job.

❖ Quality of intimacy

Physical intimacy between partners suffers greatly when either one or both people in the relationship are overweight and/or ill due to their poor diet.

Dr Lebo

Chapter 7

Who controls what you eat?

Life has a way of contradicting our preconceived notions. I had to go through a reality-check and a moment of realization. Having graduated from one of the most prestigious schools in the United States, I assumed that "I knew it all", and I was ready to come back home and make a positive impact in my country. Little did I know that I was actually just at the beginning of a life-long journey of learning. No amount of studying can replace the value of real-life practice and experience on the ground. This reality hit me when I was attending to an elderly woman from one of the remote villages in Botswana. She was admitted to Princess Marina Hospital due to complications related to uncontrolled diabetes. I was crammed full of knowledge, but I had no idea how to translate the complex technical English terms into simple Setswana to communicate effectively with my patient. I had never felt so lost in my life!

What was even more frustrating was that I could not recommend the diet I believed to be best for her, as it included foods that she had never heard of and certainly wouldn't be able to afford upon her discharge. How do you even tell someone who does not have the luxury of choice to avoid certain foods? I couldn't allow this poor elderly lady to starve for the purpose of controlling her blood sugar. Ethically and professionally, I knew that whatever recommendations I made to the patient and her family would not be easy ones. Unfortunately (or fortunately), this patient was discharged to another primary hospital to make room for sicker patients before I was required to deliver my recommendations.

I felt relieved that I had avoided having to make a difficult decision regarding this patient. If I look back, that experience prompted me to make a conscious decision to relearn what I thought I knew in the field of dietetics to incorporate an understanding of diet and nutrition within the context of my people, their culture, and even their language: Setswana. As much as I gave of my expertise to every patient I attended, interacting with each of these people was a learning experience for me. Through my clients I was able to understand what they eat, why they eat it, and their mindset towards food. I must admit that this change of approach had a completely positive impact on my growth, both professionally and personally. I evolved beyond dietician and nutritionist, into a public educator.

Every time I attended to an individual, I knew that I was really attending to the entire family unit… and even to their entire community. For example, when I would make recommendations to a Social Worker that a client should receive a food basket, I knew that, more likely than not, the rationing would not last as it would be shared among many other family members. As much as this was frustrating, especially in cases when I was trying to treat a malnourished child, I had to put my personal feelings aside. I had to do what I had to do without being judgemental. In the worst instances, I had to deal with obviously abusive family environments where certain family members would exchange food rations meant for the children for alcohol or other items. I realized that while efforts were being made to feed our communities, members within these communities were not onboard. Certainly, their mindset toward food, diet, and nutrition was extremely poor.

Early in my career as a dietitian in Botswana, I became aware that there are a lot of complex family dynamics I had to learn to understand (and sometimes just to accept) despite my personal beliefs and feelings. Whether or not this was the right decision on my part, I must admit that acceptance made my job a lot less stressful. I had to accept that things are the way they are and that I cannot change people's mindsets all the time, no matter how hard I try. Since the days of my training, I have known that making changes to one's health is a personal decision. As much as the family can be there to offer support, the patient suffering from a health condition has to take complete charge of their health with regards to their dietary habits.

Quite often, when consulting with a patient who is a married man, for example, I have found that the wife would be more knowledgeable about the patient's condition, medications, and other important information than the patient himself. If I directed any diet-related questions at the patient himself, he would mostly respond that it is not a man's job to know what food is prepared since that is the role of a woman. I had to accept that whoever was responsible for food preparation in most households was basically directly affecting their family's health status. This was a reality that I had to accept. Nevertheless, it is important to acknowledge that our socio-cultural preferences and practices greatly influence our health, and the health of our nation at large. The undeniable truth is that most people leave their health in the hands of the few who decide what they eat, when they eat, and how much is to be eaten. This is especially true in most African households.

Nowadays, with both parents working or in single-parent households, it is often the helper or the maid who prepares the meals and chooses what to cook based on the availability of food. To be honest, they often cook what is easiest, paying no attention to the amount of oil, salt, and other additives put into the food during cooking. Without guidance on what to cook and how to prepare healthy meals, domestic helpers cannot be expected to prepare balanced, nutritious meals. If, for whatever reason, one member of the family decides to go on a weight loss diet, it is often conceptualized as an individual effort without trying to change the unhealthy eating habits of the family.

I usually emphasize the importance of implementing dietary changes for the whole family, even if it is often only the mother who comes to my office to join a weight loss program. I must admit that I feel that my job has had a very positive impact even on the family members of the clients who visit my clinic, even though only one representative of that family unit has sought dietary consultation. One of the greatest concerns my clients generally have upon enrolling for the weight loss program is how they will cope when attending social events like funerals and weddings. I must admit that even as a professional dietitian, I am myself well aware that such temptations are very difficult to overcome. Weddings are the most challenging because the portions are often very large or even offered in a buffet with the expectation that guests should eat indulgently.

Meat is served as the main dish at wedding events, and is prepared such that guests will invariably have various types of meat on one plate, from stews, to fried or pounded meat (seswaa). Those preparing the food find themselves in a particularly difficult position because they have most likely sampled the dishes several times even before the invited guests eat. At funerals, even though what is served is not as varied, meat still takes center stage in the meals. What is particularly challenging at funerals is that food is most often served in the early morning. If you are someone who attends these kinds of events almost every weekend, eating healthily would definitely be a challenge.

During the Covid 19 restrictions, for obvious reasons, eating at funerals or attending social events was a luxury. During this time, healthy lunch packs consisting of fruits and sandwiches were often served at these events. Unfortunately, after the restrictions were lifted, we went back to our previous ways of doing things in excess. According to my observations, we have gone overboard with the food served at social events. It's as if we are on a mission to make up for all the lost time. It is difficult to avoid unhealthy eating, especially when food prepared away from home because one does not have control over what is offered.

My role as a Nutritionist is to educate the public about making better eating choices even in difficult situations. I resist telling people to avoid certain foods altogether, rather teaching them how to eat better by making healthy choices and being mindful about what they eat. Ultimately, my take-home message for this chapter (if it was not obvious) is that you need to take control of what you eat and be as involved in the preparation of your own food as possible. After all, what you eat concerns your health and future: you ought to be invested in the preparation and mindful consumption of every meal you partake in.

Chapter 8

Journey to Wellness

My clinical practice is based in a hospital. One particular advantages of this location is that I have the opportunity to review a wide range of medical cases referred on to me from different specialists. I interact with a diverse spectrum of clients on a daily basis, each with different medical conditions. Within the hospital where my clinic is based, there are practitioners who specialize in oncology (cancer treatment), nephrology (kidney dialysis), orthopedics (related to bones and joints), critical or intensive care, gynecology (related to diseases that affect females or their reproductive system), urology (specilizing in diseases that affect urinary system), pediatrics (related to conditions that affect children), and internal medicine (which covers a wide range of conditions affecting the internal organs of the body). In my profession, I am priviledged to be able to have access to, and the opportunity to learn from, such a wide range of medical specialists as this enables me to constantly better my skills as a clinical dietitian when it comes to managing different conditions. After years of experience dealing with a wide range of patients, I now tend to know which issues need to be addressed in what way.

As a practitioner, it is most challenging to work with patients who have gone through surgery, whether minor or major. These patients usually experience quite a lot of pain either before or after these surgeries, and they are (understandably) most interested in a "quick fix" to get rid of this pain. Patients are often referred to me from the orthopedic specialists when these patients are experiencing back problems due to excess body weight. Unfortunately, the client is more focused on immediate pain relief rather than focusing on the underlying cause of their pain - which is usually weight gain. While these patients are referred to me so that I can help them with a weight loss program, they are usually hesitant to sign up and often conclude that the referring specialist does not know what they are doing. The bottom line is that some patients are only interested in the easy route and would prefer it if some complex medical solution to their aches and pains. Committing to a dietary plan feels is too much hard work for some patients, which makes it quite a challenging to deal with them. I end up having to spend a lot of time counseling these clients, rather than discussing focusing on implementing dietary regimen or treatment plans that would support their recovery.

If you have experienced surgery yourself, especially if you are just coming out from one, I want to encourage you to be bold enough and patient enough to consider a dietary regimen as part of your treatment plan. As you deal with excess weight, you will improve the healing process. This is not an overnight process and there are no shortcuts to recovery. In fact, if you cut corners with your post-surgery healing - and most importantly, if you pay no attention to your diet and nutrition - then you are bound to wind up back in a hospital bed with a secondary disease that results from poor diet.

There are certain nutritional interventions that may assist you during post-surgery recovery and help to avoid future complications. Whether you undergo back surgery or a more common type of surgery, such as a cesarean (for women giving birth), the foods one eats in the days, weeks, and months after the procedure will affect healing and recovery. Eating the right foods can help prevent post-surgery complications, such as constipation, high blood sugar (glucose), and infections. The idea post-surgery diet differs among patients depending on the type of surgery they have had as well as any health conditions they have. A dietician will be able to help you determine the best diet to support your recovery after surgery or hospitalization.

To elaborate, if one has had a surgery that affects the bowel, a low-fiber diet may be necessary to give your digestive system a chance to heal. Every patient should make it a goal to get most of their nutrition from whole foods, rather than foods that have been heavily processed. Processed foods tend to have a lot of sugar, salt, and additives and less fiber and vitamins than their whole-food counterparts. Processed foods also contribute to inflammation, which could slow your healing process. Eating whole foods supports our overall health. With this said, one's recovery post-surgery could provide an opportunity to make long-term improvements to your eating habits. While an adverse health condition might have forced you onto a healthy diet, you may as well take advantage of the change and make it a lasting lifestyle choice that includes mindful eating and well-thought nutritional intake.

There are several medical complications that are common after any surgery. One such complication is constipation. Constipation can occur after any procedure, although it is most common after surgeries performed on the digestive tract. Many of the pain medications prescribed after surgery decrease bowel movements, leaving you constipated. Constipation can reduce one's appetite, increase pain levels, and place stress on surgical incisions. All these side-effects can undermine the healing process. It is likely that you may not feel like eating much after surgery. If you experience nausea or other symptoms, you may not want to eat at all. Your appetite should return within a few days, but it's important that you continue nourishing yourself as best you can in the meantime. Eating plenty of nourishing foods after surgery helps your body recover, supports wound healing, and prevents constipation. With all that said, you should check with your healthcare provider whether there are specific rules about what you can and cannot eat while you're recovering from a procedure.

In general, focus on eating whole foods and avoid foods that do not offer much nutrition. These are dietary choices that will support your health whether you're recovering from surgery or not (although eating healthily is especially important post-surgery. No matter how successful your surgical procedure is, your body will be working hard to heal afterwards and you can support it by consuming nutritious food. Certain foods contain nutrients that give your body the energy it needs to recover, strengthen your immune system, and help alleviate post-surgery side effects. Some foods even directly aid in healing damaged tissue and wounds.

Disclaimer: *While this book provides general tips that can be helpful, they won't apply to everyone and to all situations. Please make sure that you follow the instructions given to you by your health care professional, including your dietitian if you have been referred to one.*

Chapter 9

Diet therapy does help!

I have vivid memories from my early career days while working at Princess Marina Hospital during the height of the HIV/AIDS pandemic. The workload was so overwhelming that my time was filled up simply by patient referrals from the doctors. I never had any free time within the working day and the influx of patients was huge as a result of the pandemic. Due to my limited work experience at that time, I largely felt ill-equipped to assist these patients. Most of the patients had various nutritional complications related to advanced AIDS, such as wasting syndrome (excess weight loss and nutritional deficit), severe diarrhea, or lack of appetite or vomiting caused by Tuberculosis.

Back then, I would use a patient's weight to gauge if they were recovering, even though I did not know at the time when to stop these weight changes, especially after a patient had stabilized on Antiretroviral therapy. What I learned though, was that without sound nutritional interventions (even with medical treatment), patients took longer to recover. There is scientific evidence that nutritional interventions significantly improve outcomes in patients with chronic conditions and reduce the length of hospital stay as well as long-term complications.

While I was not conducting a controlled scientific study and collecting data, my clinical observations suggest to me that adequate nutritional intake greatly assisted the recovery of HIV positive patients on Antiretroviral therapy. Many private companies often came to the hospital to market various nutritional supplements to support patient recovery. I have no problem with this, but I have always felt that it is much simpler and much more effective to focus on eating wholesome foods. Over complicated "quick fixes" are one of the biggest problems in the field of diet and nutrition, and to be quite frank they have become a substantial societal issue. We are a people in love with

86

the instant gratification of microwaves rather than the intentional process of 'slow-cooking'. We love shortcuts and are not prepared to walk the long road. Quick fix products may offer some benefits, but due to very limited research, it is not possible for me to offer more than a personal opinion on the efficacy of such products. Do they really work? Or are they a fallacy taking advantage of the public's desperation to be healthier and to lose weight?

As a healthcare practitioner, I am regulated by and held accountable to the laws and standards of Botswana. It is my responsibility to serve the best interests of the public, not to mislead them. Sometimes clients tell me that they expect me to validate or endorse certain information that they have heard or read elsewhere that makes recommendations of how to manage or prevent certain conditions. It is surprising to me that most clients go to the hospital with the intention of getting a professional medical diagnosis, but then they deny diagnosis and medical advice they are given in favor of alternative therapies. Don't get me wrong, there is a place for alternative therapies, but they shouldn't be used as a means to put off doing the necessary lifestyle work to manage their conditions. If you are reading this book and you have an underlying condition, I humbly implore you to follow the advice of healthcare professionals and to choose scientifically-based medical interventions that offer you the best chance of overall improvement. Alternative therapies are poorly regulated and conclusive studies have not been conducted regarding their side effects or their effectiveness in treating your condition.

Even if you accept a medical diagnosis, opting for an alternative treatment is a risky way of managing it. For example, I've had clients who have been diagnosed with conditions as serious as kidney failure who require much convincing before they agree to incorporate the diet therapy that is recommended as medical best practice. My years of experience have taught me that it is these types of patients that are most likely to accuse me of malpractice because they are unwilling to accept that certain medical protocols are required to manage chronic illnesses. They would most likely have already been told by another dietitian or health care professional what they need to do, but instead they go into denial and come to me looking for a second opinion - only to be given the same advice. In all honesty, these patients are desperately searching for someone to endorse their preference for alternative therapies.

I admit that it is not easy coming to terms with a diagnosis of chronic illness, especially in the early days. I am well aware of the fear and anxiety that one goes through upon diagnosis. The required lifestyle changes and a dependence on medicine can be very overwhelming. In my experience, a doctor will always advise their patients to make lifestyle or dietary changes before they start prescribing medications. This is especially typical in the case of pre-diabetic patients. These patients often take these initial lifestyle recommendations lightly and do not make any effort to implement them until it's too late. Generally, by the time these people are referred to a dietitian, such as myself, they have already reached the point where they are required to be on medications and dietary changes have become a prescription, rather than advice.

I acknowledge that many patients face the very real difficulty of financial constraints, among others. Some clients will mention that they can only afford that which is what is commonly available. At the end of the day, however, dieticians are still held accountable for doing their job. This is very challenging professionally: what does one do when dealing with a client who faces these challenges? Scientifically, I know that it is possible for clients diagnosed with certain conditions to come off their medications once they are receiving controlled, carefully monitored diet therapy. Unfortunately, a client who has limited resources may not be able to adhere to the dietary recommendations that enable such improvements. This reality is by far one of the most challenging issues with my professional context.

In other cases I merely educate people about their conditions in order for them to gain the confidence to self-monitor their condition - for example, diabetes. The greatest difficulty for most of my diabetic patients is not necessarily following a meal plan, but rather believing that they are able to manage their condition themselves. Diabetes is one of the most common, yet misunderstood, conditions in our society. Most clients who are referred to me to help them manage their condition lack confidence in their ability to do so and feel disempowered by their diagnosis. It takes time to build their trust, both in me and in themselves. Their treatment requires a mindset shift in which they come to understand that diet therapy is the secret to successfully managing the condition that they have been made to believe will kill them. Yes, there can be severe complications associated with diabetes, such as blindness, kidney, and heart disease, and even the need for limb amputation. Nevertheless, the solution to diabetes is relatively simple: control your blood sugar levels.

Most clients who are referred to a dietitian are shocked when they find out that they can actually monitor their blood sugar and therefore manage their diabetes through diet. I explain to them that using medical treatments, such as tablets or insulin injections, does not protect them from their diabetes and allow them to eat what they want. If they were to take this approach it would only be a matter of time before serious complications arise. What if I told you that it is very possible for you to live your life off medications altogether... you can in fact live a life completely independent of them! Knowing this, what will you do? Would you be willing to make the necessary lifestyle and dietary changes?

Dr Lebo

Chapter 10

Just do it

A stumbling block for many people wishing to change their diet is knowing where to start. You may have no idea how much a new diet will cost or worry that some of the necessary foods may be unavailable to you. It is easy to become overwhelmed when pursuing anything that we don't routinely do. Change of any kind pushes us out of our comfort zone, and this is difficult. Most people are so used to buying the same foods from the same grocery stores around the same time of the week or month. Making a total shift requires patience and discipline. Here are a few practical and simple handles to follow:

- Follow **an eating plan**: More often than not, people buy what they think they will need while doing their groceries, rather than making purchases according to a clear meal plan. Once you know what a healthy diet is, this considerably eases the stress of trying to figure out what to eat. Try to begin your dietary changes by following a weekly eating or diet plan. An **eating plan** outlines what you will eat throughout the day. It includes your breakfast, lunch, dinner, drinks, and any snacks. An eating plan could help one budget for specific foods, identify nutritional excesses and deficiencies in their diet, and minimize mindless eating. It is common practice for most people to buy what is available without prior planning or to end up eating compulsively at restaurants. One is less likely to fall into these traps when following a meal plan however.

- **<u>Cycle meal plans weekly:</u>** It is also advisable to **cycle your meal plans so that you are following a different meal plan each week.** This helps to avoid monotony and enables one to better budget for less commonplace foods, such as seasonal fruits and vegetables. One can also start a collection of recipes in order to make the preparation of healthy food easier. These recipes should avoid salt, sugar, and fat. Following a meal plan can also help the rest of the family, especially family members with varied nutritional and needs and eating preferences. Children are less likely to refuse certain foods if they know what to expect on specific days, rather than being surprised at meal time. Another benefit of good meal planning is that you will come to know where to get the best possible fresh fruits and vegetables, and even traditional grains and pulses. Many pop-up markets sell a wide variety of traditional foods that are not stocked in grocery stores.

- **<u>Involve children in planning and preparing their own meals:</u>** One of the challenges that parents face is having to pack meals for the children to eat at school. It is tricky to know what to pack, especially if you want to provide them with healthy food items. This dilemma is greatly eased by having a meal plan that you use for easy-to-prepare school lunches. Try to involve your children in the preparation of their meals. They could do something as simple as cutting their own fruit (under close supervision), or you could encourage them to assist you while you cook. There are a number of simple recipes that are child-friendly. Involving children in cooking and food preparation can help them learn important skills, like teamwork, reading, and following sequential instructions. Parents hardly ever involve their children when they go grocery shopping, but shopping is an opportunity to help your children learn about budgeting and healthy foods. This can be a fun experience for them that moreover teaches them to appreciate different foods.

- **Know the suggested portion sizes for your children (and other household members):** Once your children appreciate the cost of buying food, they may also learn how to establish a healthy relationship with food by controlling portion sizes. This is important because we are increasingly experiencing childhood obesity as a societal issue. I often hear parents complaining that their children binge on fruit drinks and bread when these items are in the house, and that they then do not want to eat other more nutritious foods that are prepared for them at home. Parents also sometimes complain that when they pack healthy school lunches for their children, there is always wastage as most of it returns with them from school. It really helps when children know ahead of time what is packed in their lunch boxes and when they are involved in packing their school lunches. If they are included in the decision-making and lunch-packing process, they are more likely to eat it. Just as with family meals, a meal plan for school lunches is very important. These meal plans not only help with budgeting, but also provide parents with ideas of healthy snacks and beverages that they can prepare for their children.

I cannot emphasize this enough: know your child's recommended portion limits. Parents often make the mistake of dishing up more food for their children than their bodies can actually process within healthily. Children do not always eat the same portion sizes on a daily basis, therefore it is very important to also consider how much food they actually want when dishing up for them. Honoring your child's awareness of their own body by not forcing them to finish a helping of food that may be too much for their small bodies also builds a sense of ownership, responsibility, and an understanding of portion control within them. This is true not only for children but even for the adults in the household. It tends to be common practice for the cook to dish up food for everyone, but it can help to avoid food waste and over-eating if each person dishes up for themselves only how much they want. As family members practice dishing up for themselves, each of them will eventually learn not to over-dish, especially if they know that the rest of the members haven't eaten yet.

- **<u>Food preparation is key:</u>** Healthy eating is not just about avoiding junk food and large portions. Sometimes, healthy food can be made unhealthy based on the way we prepare our food (combining them with other unhealthy ingredients or using unhealthy cooking methods). For example, spinach can be made unhealthy by cooking it with a lot of spices, oil, or even cream (this is how some people prepare creamed spinach). Spinach is very nutritious, but when one adds these other unhealthy ingredients the resultant spinach dish becomes very high in calories and even salt in salt content.

- **<u>Read food labels:</u>** Even though it may be challenging initially, one should make healthy choices at the grocery store by always reading (and understanding) the labels on food items before buying them. As you start to read labels you may find that you wish to avoid some of the cheaper food items, or food items that you used to commonly buy, due to the unhealthy additives or ingredients that they contain. If someone in the household has a medical condition, such as allergies or diabetes, it is especially necessary to read food labels as this practice will help you avoid buying foods that contain ingredients that could aggravate these medical conditions. Even though fruit and vegetables are not labeled, it is important to include these in your diet and vary them as much as possible. The produce that is in-season is usually cheaper and more widely available. For example, during a certain time of the year, corn and watermelon are widely available. Plan your meals around what is available at the time.

- Avoid **<u>overconsumption, even of nutritious foods:</u>** A healthy diet is not only about what one eats, but how much one eats of a particular food. Sometimes people can eat too much of a nutritious food. Meat consumption is a common example of this. It is the norm for many people to eat meat with almost every meal (especially lunches and suppers). Yes, meat is nutritious, but overconsumption of meat can contribute to conditions, such as gout and heart issues. Because of our societal tendency to over consume meat, I have started a "Meatless Monday" campaign that I promote through my social media platform. When I first started providing health education around Meatless Monday, I got a lot of backlash from some members of the public. These people felt that I had no right to dictate to them how they should eat the food they buy with their own money, and that they should be allowed the freedom to eat what they want, when they want, and how they want. It is true that everyone does have this right. My role is not to dictate to you, but to provide you with the knowledge to (hopefully) make choices that will benefit your longevity and well-being. It took a couple of weeks of sharing educational content around the benefits of skipping meat just once a week before my following started to join in. Before launching the Meatless Monday campaign, I must acknowledge that I was actually eating meat on Mondays. But because I always want to practice what I preach, I started implementing the Meatless Monday practice in my own life as soon as I launched the campaign. I have since been amazed by the benefits I have experienced from simply not eating meat once a week.

An unintentional result of my Meatless Monday habit has been that I have reduced the amount of meat that I consume the rest of the week too. My Meatless Monday made me aware that I could get the same nutrients that I get from meat, by eating other healthier foods, like certain types of beans. Not only has my life been transformed by Meatless Monday, but I have had overwhelming feedback from other members of the public, both via my social media platform and in person, about how this simple habit has changed their health. They achieved these benefits without really "knowing" what they were doing, and simply by following the Meatless Monday challenge instructions.

My social media account has the intention of providing people with the information they need to become educated on diet and nutrition. I do my best to also provide my followers with tools that will enable them to take control of their health. Meatless Monday is just one example of a healthy practice I have shared on social media. I also share other health recommendations, such as drinking water ('every sip counts') and controlling portion size (by using a 'bikiri' or cup to measure out advisable portion sizes). While these suggestions are simple, I have found that many people in my following have needed them. The sheer volume of positive testimonies that I receive makes the efficacy of these practices undeniable. Members of the public have sent me testimonies describing how they have been able to fall pregnant, that they are experiencing better skin, or improved blood pressure (to mention a few) since participating in my challenges and following my online advice.

I must disclaim that I do not know the people who send me these testimonies and I have not personally verified their legitimacy. Nonetheless, the feedback continues to stream in with people telling me everyday how they had given up on a particular health condition but how they are now taking charge of their health and feeling excited about the future. I believe that it is important to empower everyone, regardless of their background or socio-economic status. Please understand that you do not have to eat "fancy" or expensive foods to eat healthily. While the advice offered in this book cannot compare to that offered in a personalized medical consultation - either with myself, another dietician, or some other healthcare professional - I encourage you to implement some of the dietary and lifestyle changes that it has suggested, even before you seek consultation with a dietitian. As every person has individualized needs, and may additionally have certain medical conditions that need to be addressed, tailor-made programs are most effective in catering to these specific needs and addressing issues. To avoid potentially harmful outcomes, please be sure to work with a qualified (and registered) professional if you choose to seek dietary consultation.

Ultimately, I hope you become THE MINDFUL EATER you ought to be!

Dr Lebo

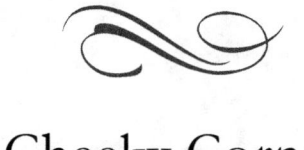

Cheeky Corner

Grumbling stomach? Do you really need to eat or it is your system stretching?

*****

Bored? Food is not for entertainment... go for a walk!

*****

Everything that goes into your mouth is by choice: choose wisely

*****

Your body is not a rubbish bin!

*****

What you eat today determines what diseases you will have tomorrow.

*****

You need nutrients, not food! Eat quality not quantity.

*****

The number on the scale reflects how much you eat.

*****

Be mindful. Don't forget what you have eaten, how much you have eaten, and why you ate it in the first place.

You can't have your cake and eat it!

*****

Aging is a disease. Nourishing your body will delay it.

Acknowledgements

One of the things I have learned in life is to value those very close to my heart, and that is my family. Without their support, I would definitely not be where I am today. My deepest gratitude goes out to my husband, Benjamin, who has put up with my long working hours, especially during the time that I was furthering my studies, and now while writing this book. He has been an incredible 'double parent', ever-present to our children, Leatile and Reneiloe, when I could not be there for them. My parents, Michael Motshidi and Janet Spivey, have always valued education even though they were not educated as children. They supported all of their children, including me, through our education and encouraged us to never give up. I am indebted to them for raising the woman I am today. Lastly, I want to immensely thank Lazarus Takawira for convincing me to write this book even though I was reluctant and full of all sorts of excuses not to! However, his persistence is why this resource exists today. I hope that it will greatly benefit all who will read it.

About the Author

Dr. Malebɔgo Eluya is a wife, mother, daughter, and has been a Registered Dietician and Nutritionist with the Botswana Health Professions Council since 2001. Affectionately known as "Dr. Lebo" to the general public, she is largely associated with the #MeatlessMonday challenge designed to encourage the public to change their attitude towards healthy eating through mindfulness. Dr. Lebo studied a Bachelor of Science Degree in Nutritional Sciences at Howard University in the United States of America. After graduating, she decided to relocate back to Botswana to serve her country. She spent more than a decade working with the Botswana Defence Force before receiving an opportunity to pursue a Master of Science Degree in International Public Health Nutrition at Westminster University in the United Kingdom. While studying this degree, Dr. Lebo's passion for preventative diet therapy was fueled. As someone who appreciates a challenge, she made a career move into academia, where she pursued a Doctorate of Philosophy in Human Nutrition at a tertiary institution in South Africa, while running a private clinic on the side. After remaining in academia for a little over five years, Dr. Lebo took a leap of faith and directed her attention to run her clinic full-time. She made this change in 2020, at the height of the Covid 19 pandemic. With no clients able to visit the clinic, Dr. Lebo began using social media as a platform to educate the public. This turned out to be an unforeseen blessing for Dr. Lebo's clinic as well, unexpectedly boosting its business. With this book, Dr. Lebo hopes to continue inspiring people to pursue healthy living, or even run their own businesses!

The Mindful Eater!!!

www.ingramcontent.com/pod-product-compliance
Lightning Source LLC
Chambersburg PA
CBHW060405290526
45791CB00002B/609